THE NO GALLBLADDER DIET COOKBOOK FOR SENIORS

A Comprehensive Guide to Eating Well, Supporting Digestive Health, and Savoring Every Bite After Gallbladder Surgery | 7 Day Meal Plan Included

Rosie K. Bratt

TABLE OF CONTENT

INTRODUCTION
CHAPTER 1
CHAPTER 2
CHAPTER 3
CHAPTER 4
CHAPTER 5
CHAPTER 6
CHAPTER 7
CHAPTER 8
CHAPTER 9
CHAPTER 10
CONCLUSION

INTRODUCTION

Welcome to our journey to better health and well-being, designed specifically for our beloved seniors. As we age gracefully, our bodies undergo various changes, and one vital organ that frequently requires our attention is the gallbladder. This introduction serves as a guiding light, illuminating the path to understanding, nurturing, and nourishing your gallbladder health through the power of a well-planned diet.

About the Gallbladder: An Overview

The gallbladder is a small but powerful organ located beneath the liver that plays an important role in our digestive system. Its primary function is to store and concentrate bile, a digestive fluid produced by the liver to aid in the breakdown of fats. When we eat fatty or greasy foods, the gallbladder contracts and releases bile into the small intestine, allowing us to digest and absorb essential nutrients.

The Importance of Diet for Gallbladder Health

In the intricate dance of digestive harmony, diet plays a critical role. What we eat has a direct impact on the health and function of our gallbladder. A diet high in unhealthy fats, processed foods, and high cholesterol can strain the gallbladder, causing discomfort, inflammation, and potentially serious conditions like gallstones or gallbladder disease.

How Does Aging Affect the Gallbladder

Our bodies change naturally as we age, which can have an impact on the gallbladder's efficiency and resilience. Metabolic processes may slow, digestion may become less efficient, and certain medical conditions or medications commonly associated with aging can increase the risk of gallbladder problems in seniors. Seniors must take proactive steps to maintain gallbladder health through mindful dietary and lifestyle choices.

The advantages of a gallbladder-friendly diet for seniors

Starting a gallbladder-friendly diet has numerous advantages for seniors looking to improve their health and vitality:

1. Relieving Discomfort: By eating foods that are gentle on the gallbladder, seniors can reduce their risk of digestive discomfort, bloating, and pain associated with gallbladder problems.

2. Preventing Complications: A gallbladder-friendly diet can help prevent the formation of gallstones and lower the risk of developing gallbladder disease, reducing the need for invasive medical interventions.

3. Promoting Nutritional Wellness: By focusing on nutrient-dense, whole foods, seniors can ensure they are getting the vitamins, minerals, and antioxidants they need for good health and vitality.

4. Improving Quality of Life: Proper gallbladder health leads to better digestion, more energy, and a greater sense of well-being, allowing seniors to fully embrace and enjoy their golden years.

In this Gallbladder Diet Cookbook for Seniors, we'll go on a culinary adventure full of delicious, nourishing recipes, practical tips, and expert advice to help you nourish your gallbladder while also nurturing your overall health and vitality. Allow this cookbook to be your trusted companion as you strive for optimal gallbladder health, one delectable dish at a time.

This introduction sets the stage by providing seniors with a thorough understanding of the gallbladder, the role of diet in maintaining its health, and the special considerations that come with aging. It aims to inspire and empower seniors to take control of their health through mindful dietary choices and lifestyle habits, laying the groundwork for the transformative journey that awaits them within the pages of the cookbook.

CHAPTER 1

The Gallbladder Basics

In the complex landscape of human anatomy, the gallbladder is a small but vital organ that plays an important role in the digestive process. This chapter is a foundational cornerstone, delving deeply into the anatomy, function, and common disorders of the gallbladder, providing readers with the necessary knowledge to navigate the complexities of gallbladder health.

1.1 Anatomy and Function of Gallbladder

The gallbladder, a pear-shaped organ located beneath the liver, may be small, but its importance cannot be overstated. The gallbladder serves as a reservoir for bile, a vital digestive fluid produced by the liver, and is essential for the breakdown and absorption of dietary fats. When we eat fatty foods, the gallbladder contracts and releases bile into the small intestine, emulsifying fats and allowing them to be digested and absorbed into the bloodstream.

A thorough examination of the gallbladder's anatomy reveals its complex structure, including the cystic duct, which connects it to the common bile duct and facilitates bile flow into the digestive tract. Understanding the anatomy of the gallbladder provides invaluable insight into its function and the intricate interplay of physiological processes that support optimal digestion.

1.2: Common Gallbladder Disorders in Seniors

Despite its resilience, the gallbladder is vulnerable to a variety of disorders and conditions that can disrupt its function and jeopardize digestive health, particularly in the elderly. The most common gallbladder disorders are:

- **Gallstones:** Hardened deposits of bile components that can clog the bile ducts, causing pain, inflammation, and other complications.

- **Cholecystitis:** Gallbladder inflammation, usually caused by gallstones or infection, resulting in severe abdominal pain, fever, and nausea.

- **Biliary Dyskinesia:** Impaired gallbladder motility causes dysfunction and digestive disturbances in the absence of gallstones.

- **Gallbladder Cancer:** Although uncommon, gallbladder cancer can occur, especially in seniors with a history of gallbladder disease or chronic inflammation.

Seniors can prevent complications by becoming familiar with the signs, symptoms, and risk factors associated with these conditions.

1.3 Symptoms and Signs of Gallbladder Disorders

Recognizing the subtle cues and warning signs of gallbladder dysfunction is critical for early detection and treatment. Common symptoms of gallbladder issues in seniors can include:

- **Abdominal Pain:** Persistent pain in the upper right abdomen that frequently radiates to the back or shoulder blades, particularly after high-fat meals.
- **Nausea and Vomiting:** Feelings of nausea accompanied by vomiting or indigestion, especially after eating fatty foods.
- **Digestive Disturbances:** Bloating, gas, diarrhea, or constipation could indicate gallbladder dysfunction.
- **Jaundice:** Yellowing of the skin and eyes caused by impaired bile flow, which may indicate a bile duct blockage.

Seniors can prevent further complications by paying attention to these warning signs and seeking medical attention as soon as possible.

1.4: Diagnosis and Treatment Options

In the quest for gallbladder health, accurate diagnosis and tailored treatment strategies are critical. Ultrasound, CT scans, and blood tests allow healthcare providers to evaluate gallbladder function, identify abnormalities, and develop personalized treatment plans.

Treatment options for gallbladder disorders can vary depending on the nature and severity of the condition, ranging from conservative measures like dietary changes and medications to surgical interventions like cholecystectomy. Seniors are encouraged to communicate openly with their healthcare providers about treatment options that meet their specific needs and preferences, fostering a collaborative approach to gallbladder care.

By delving into the fundamentals of gallbladder anatomy, function, disorders, and diagnostic approaches, Chapter 1 provides seniors with the knowledge and insight they need to embark on a journey to optimal gallbladder health. With this understanding, readers are able to confidently and clearly navigate the complexities of gallbladder health, laying the groundwork for transformative dietary and lifestyle interventions discussed in later chapters.

This chapter gives seniors a thorough understanding of the gallbladder, including its function, common disorders, symptoms, and diagnostic and treatment options, allowing them to manage their gallbladder health and make informed decisions in collaboration with healthcare providers.

CHAPTER 2

The Senior's Guide to a Gallbladder-Friendly Diet

Diet is a cornerstone in the intricate tapestry of digestive health, having a significant impact on gallbladder function and well-being. This chapter serves as a compass, guiding seniors through the principles, practices, and dietary considerations required to maintain gallbladder health and promote digestive harmony in their golden years.

2.1 Principles of the Gallbladder Diet

A gallbladder-friendly diet emphasizes balance, moderation, and mindfulness, with a focus on foods that promote optimal digestion while reducing gallbladder stress. The key principles include:

- Moderate Fat Intake: While fat is an essential nutrient, seniors should choose healthy fats like avocados, nuts, seeds, and fatty fish, while limiting saturated and trans fats from processed and fried foods.

- Embrace Fiber-Rich Foods: High-fiber foods like fruits, vegetables, whole grains, and legumes promote regularity and help with waste elimination, lowering the risk of gallstones.

- Prioritize Lean Proteins: Seniors should consume lean protein sources such as poultry, fish, tofu, and legumes while avoiding fatty cuts of meat and processed meats.

- Stay Hydrated: Adequate hydration is required to maintain bile fluidity and promote optimal digestion. Seniors should drink plenty of water throughout the day, supplemented with herbal teas and hydrating foods like fruits and vegetables.

- Portion Control: Seniors should eat mindfully, focusing on smaller, more frequent meals to avoid overloading the gallbladder and reducing digestive discomfort.

By following these guiding principles, seniors can cultivate a dietary approach that nourishes the gallbladder, promotes digestive health, and improves overall well-being.

2.2: Foods to Include and Avoid

Shopping with gallbladder health in mind requires discernment and awareness. Seniors should incorporate the following gallbladder-friendly foods into their diets:

- **Fruits and Vegetables:** Fruits and vegetables are high in fiber, vitamins, and antioxidants, making them essential components of a gallbladder-friendly diet. Seniors should consume a diverse range of produce, such as leafy greens, berries, citrus fruits, and cruciferous vegetables.

- **Whole Grains:** Whole grains, such as oats, quinoa, brown rice, and whole wheat, provide sustained energy and promote digestive health due to their high fiber content.
- **Healthy Fats:** Including sources of healthy fats like olive oil, avocado, nuts, and seeds in meals adds flavor and satiety without overburdening the gallbladder.
- **Lean Proteins:** Seniors should prioritize lean protein sources like skinless poultry, fish, tofu, and legumes, while limiting their intake of red meat and processed meats high in saturated fat.
- **Hydration:** Water is the elixir of life, necessary for proper hydration and digestive function. Seniors should aim to drink at least 8-10 glasses of water per day, with intake adjusted based on personal needs and activity levels.

Conversely, certain foods may exacerbate gallbladder symptoms and should be consumed sparingly or avoided entirely, including:

- **Fried and Fatty Foods:** Consuming greasy, fried foods and dishes high in saturated and trans fats can cause gallbladder pain and digestive discomfort.
- **Processed Foods:** Highly processed foods, such as sugary snacks, refined grains, and convenience meals, are frequently devoid of nutrients and can cause inflammation and digestive issues.
- **Spicy Foods:** For some people, spicy foods can aggravate gallbladder symptoms and should be consumed in moderation or avoided entirely, depending on tolerance levels.
- **Alcohol and Caffeine:** Seniors should consume alcohol and caffeine in moderation, as excessive consumption can dehydrate the body and exacerbate gallbladder issues.

Seniors can create a gallbladder-friendly diet by making informed choices and focusing on nutrient-dense, whole foods that nourish the body, support digestive health, and improve overall well-being.

2.3 Portion Control and Meal Timing Tip

In the quest for gallbladder health, portion control and mindful eating practices are critical in promoting optimal digestion and reducing discomfort. Senior citizens are encouraged to:

- **Eat Smaller, More Frequent Meals:** Eating smaller meals throughout the day, spaced evenly apart, can help prevent gallbladder overload and promote regular digestion.
- **Chew Thoroughly:** Chewing food slowly and thoroughly helps in the early stages of digestion, reducing the workload on the

gallbladder and reducing digestive discomfort.

- **Avoid Eating Late at Night:** Seniors should try to eat their last meal at least two to three hours before bedtime to allow for proper digestion and avoid reflux-related symptoms.

- **Listen to Your Body:** Paying attention to hunger and satiety cues allows seniors to eat intuitively, preventing overeating and promoting healthy digestion.

By implementing these portion control and meal timing strategies, seniors can improve digestive function, reduce gallbladder burden, and enjoy meals with greater comfort and satisfaction.

2.4 The Importance of Hydration

Water is the unsung hero of digestive health, contributing significantly to optimal hydration, bile production, and efficient digestion. Seniors should prioritize hydration as follows:

- **Drinking Ample Water:** Seniors should aim to drink at least 8-10 glasses of water per day, with intake adjusted based on individual needs, activity levels, and environmental factors.
- **Infusing Flavor Naturally:** Infusing water with fresh herbs, fruits, or cucumber slices adds flavor and promotes hydration without the use of sugary additives.
- **Drinking Herbal Teas:** Herbal teas like peppermint, ginger, and chamomile can soothe the digestive system, relieve discomfort, and promote relaxation.

Staying hydrated can help seniors maintain gallbladder health, promote optimal digestion, and improve overall well-being in their golden years.

Chapter 2 provides seniors with the necessary knowledge and practical strategies for cultivating a gallbladder-friendly diet that nourishes the body, promotes digestive health, and improves overall well-being. Seniors can embark on a transformative dietary journey by adopting the guiding principles of moderation, balance, and mindfulness, laying the groundwork for lifelong digestive harmony and vitality.

This chapter offers seniors practical advice on creating a gallbladder-friendly diet, including principles of healthy eating, foods to include and avoid, portion control strategies, meal timing tips, and the importance of hydration. By adopting these dietary principles and practices, seniors can improve gallbladder health, digestion, and overall well-being in their golden years.

CHAPTER 3

Preparing Balanced Meals for Gallbladder Health

In the culinary symphony of life, each meal is a harmonious blend of flavors, textures, and nutrients that nourish the body while also nurturing the spirit. This chapter acts as a culinary compass, guiding seniors through the process of creating balanced meals that promote gallbladder health, digestive harmony, and tantalize the taste buds with delectable flavors and textures.

3.1 Breakfast Ideas

Breakfast, the morning muse of culinary creativity, sets the tone for the day ahead, providing vital nourishment and energy to seniors' activities. Some gallbladder-friendly breakfast ideas include:

- **Oatmeal:** Creamy oatmeal topped with fresh berries, sliced bananas, and a sprinkle of nuts or seeds makes for a hearty and fiber-rich breakfast.

- **Greek Yogurt Parfait:** Layered Greek yogurt, granola, honey, and diced fruit make a filling and protein-packed breakfast option.
- **Vegetable Omelet:** A fluffy vegetable omelet with spinach, bell peppers, onions, and tomatoes is a savory and nutrient-dense breakfast option.

Seniors can start their day off right by incorporating protein, fiber, and healthy fats into their morning meals, which supports gallbladder health and promotes sustained energy levels.

3.2 Lunch Time Favorites

Midday meals entice seniors with a variety of delectable options, inviting them to indulge in wholesome, satisfying fare that will see them through the afternoon.

Lunchtime favorites suitable for the gallbladder include:

- **Quinoa Salad:** A colorful quinoa salad with mixed greens, cherry tomatoes, cucumbers, feta cheese, and lemon vinaigrette dressing makes for a refreshing and nutrient-dense lunch option.
- **Grilled Chicken Wrap:** A whole-grain wrap filled with grilled chicken, avocado, lettuce, tomatoes, and a drizzle of yogurt-based dressing makes for a protein-packed and portable lunch option.
- **Vegetable Soup:** A hearty vegetable soup made with carrots, celery, potatoes, and beans provides warmth and comfort on cold days while also providing essential nutrients and fiber.

Seniors who incorporate a variety of colorful vegetables, lean proteins, and whole grains into their midday meals can satisfy their hunger, support digestive health, and nourish their bodies with nutritious goodness.

3.3 Delicious Dinners

As the sun sets on another day, dinner beckons, promising culinary adventures and delights that soothe the soul and nourish the body. Gallbladder-friendly dinner options include:

- **Baked Salmon:** Succulent baked salmon seasoned with herbs and spices, served with roasted vegetables and quinoa, is a protein- and omega-3 fatty acid-rich dinner option.
- **Stir-Fried Tofu and Vegetables:** Crispy stir-fried tofu with broccoli, bell peppers, snap peas, and mushrooms served over brown rice or noodles makes a filling and plant-based dinner option.
- **Turkey Meatballs with Marinara Sauce:** Tender turkey meatballs simmered in marinara sauce, served over whole-grain

pasta or zucchini noodles, are a hearty and protein-packed dinner option.

Seniors can enjoy delicious and satisfying dinners that promote gallbladder health and overall well-being by including a variety of lean proteins, colorful vegetables, and whole grains.

3.4 Snack and Dessert

Between-meal cravings and sweet indulgences entice and delight seniors, allowing them to savor small moments of culinary joy throughout the day. Here are some gallbladder-friendly snack and dessert ideas:

- **Fruit and Nut Butter:** Sliced apples or bananas with nut butter make a filling and nutrient-dense snack option.
- **Yogurt and Berries:** For a sweet and protein-rich dessert, top creamy Greek

yogurt with fresh berries and drizzle with honey.

- **Dark Chocolate**: A square of dark chocolate (70% cocoa or higher) is a decadent and antioxidant-rich treat that will satisfy your sweet tooth without overloading your gallbladder.

Seniors can enjoy guilt-free culinary pleasures that improve their overall well-being by selecting nutrient-dense snacks and desserts that satisfy cravings while also supporting gallbladder health.

In Chapter 3, seniors are taken on a culinary journey through balanced meals, tantalizing flavors, and nourishing ingredients that promote gallbladder health and digestive balance. Seniors can enjoy the benefits of healthy eating and nourish their bodies by embracing the art of meal preparation with creativity, mindfulness, and culinary flair.

This chapter offers seniors a variety of balanced meal ideas for breakfast, lunch, and dinner, as well as snack and dessert options, all of which are intended to promote gallbladder health while tantalizing the taste buds with delicious flavors and textures. Seniors can enjoy a diverse and satisfying diet that promotes digestive harmony and improves overall well-being by including nutrient-dense ingredients and culinary creativity in their meals.

CHAPTER 4

Delicious Recipes For Gallbladder Health

Recipes act as vibrant brushstrokes on the culinary canvas of life, creating a tapestry of flavors, textures, and aromas that delight the senses and nourish the body. This chapter is a treasure trove of culinary inspiration, providing seniors with a collection of delicious recipes carefully crafted to support gallbladder health, promote digestive harmony, and tantalize the taste buds with nutritious goodness.

4.1 Appetizers and Starters

The path to culinary delight begins with delectable appetizers and starters that whet the appetite and set the tone for an unforgettable dining experience. Here are some gallbladder-friendly appetizer ideas:

- **Stuffed Mushrooms:** Baked crimini mushrooms with a savory mixture of spinach, garlic, and feta cheese, topped with fresh parsley.
- **Cucumber Avocado Rolls:** Thinly sliced cucumbers are rolled up with creamy avocado, smoked salmon, and dill for a refreshing and elegant appetizer.
- **Quinoa Salad Cups:** Miniature cups filled with a vibrant quinoa salad made with diced vegetables, fresh herbs, and a zesty lemon dressing, ideal for serving at gatherings or parties.

Seniors can stimulate their appetites, support digestion, and enjoy the anticipation of future culinary delights by beginning their meals with nutrient-rich appetizers and starters.

4.2 Soups and Salads

Soups and salads contain a variety of flavors, textures, and nutrients, providing seniors with nutritious options that satisfy hunger and promote digestive health. Here are some soup and salad recipes that are gallbladder-friendly:

- **Roasted Vegetable Soup:** This hearty soup is made with roasted carrots, sweet potatoes, onions, and garlic, blended until smooth, and garnished with Greek yogurt and fresh herbs.
- **Kale Caesar Salad:** Crisp kale leaves are tossed with homemade Caesar dressing, whole-grain croutons, and grated Parmesan cheese for a healthy twist on a classic salad favorite.
- **Chickpea and Quinoa Salad:** A protein-packed salad with chickpeas, quinoa, cherry tomatoes, cucumbers, and feta cheese, tossed in a tangy vinaigrette and topped with fresh parsley.

Seniors can enjoy satisfying and nutrient-dense meals that support gallbladder health and promote overall well-being by including a variety of vegetables, legumes, and whole grains in their soups and salads.

4.3 Main Courses

Main courses take center stage, providing seniors with a showcase of culinary creativity and gastronomic delight that satisfies hunger while also nourishing the body. Gallbladder-friendly main dish recipes include:

- **Baked Lemon Herb Chicken:** Tender chicken breasts marinated in a zesty mixture of lemon juice, garlic, and fresh herbs, then baked to perfection and served with roasted vegetables.
- **Vegetable Stir-Fry:** A colorful stir-fry with a variety of fresh vegetables, including bell peppers, broccoli, snap peas, and mushrooms, tossed in a savory sauce and served over brown rice or quinoa.

- Grilled Salmon with Mango Salsa:
Flaky grilled salmon filets are topped with a vibrant mango salsa made from diced mango, red onion, cilantro, and lime juice, providing a burst of tropical flavor with each bite.

Seniors can enjoy satisfying and nourishing meals that support gallbladder health and digestive harmony by experimenting with a variety of main course options that include lean proteins, colorful vegetables, and whole grains.

4.4 Side Dish and Accompaniment

Side dishes and accompaniments enhance the dining experience by providing complementary flavors and textures. Here are some gallbladder-friendly side dish and accompaniment recipes:

- Roasted Garlic Mashed Cauliflower:
Creamy mashed cauliflower infused with

roasted garlic, butter, and fresh herbs, serving as a flavorful and low-carb alternative to traditional mashed potatoes.

- **Quinoa Pilaf:** Fluffy quinoa cooked with diced vegetables, toasted nuts, and dried fruits, seasoned with aromatic spices, and topped with fresh parsley.

- **Balsamic Glazed Brussels Sprouts:** Tender Brussels sprouts are roasted to perfection and drizzled with a tangy balsamic glaze, creating a sweet and savory side dish that compliments any meal.

Seniors can improve the flavor and nutritional profile of their meals by incorporating nutrient-dense side dishes and accompaniments, while also supporting gallbladder health and overall well-being.

4.5 Sauces, dressings, and condiments

Sauces, dressings, and condiments add depth and complexity to dishes, boosting flavor and appeal with a burst of culinary innovation. Here are some gallbladder-friendly sauce, dressing, and condiment recipes:

- **Greek Yogurt Tzatziki Sauce:** Creamy Greek yogurt is blended with grated cucumber, garlic, dill, and lemon juice, creating a refreshing and versatile sauce for dipping or drizzling.
- **Balsamic Vinaigrette Dressing:** This tangy vinaigrette made with balsamic vinegar, olive oil, Dijon mustard, and honey is ideal for dressing salads or marinating meats and vegetables.
- **Homemade Pesto:** This vibrant pesto, made with fresh basil, pine nuts, Parmesan cheese, garlic, and olive oil, adds a burst of herbaceous flavor to pasta dishes, sandwiches, or grilled vegetables.

Seniors can control the quality of ingredients and customize flavors to suit their taste preferences by making their own sauces, dressings, and condiments, which improves meal enjoyment while also supporting gallbladder health.

4.6 Sweet Treats and Desserts

Indulgent sweet treats and desserts allow seniors to satisfy their sweet tooth while nourishing their bodies with nutritious ingredients. Here are some gallbladder-friendly sweet treat and dessert recipes:

- **Baked Apple Crisp:** Tender baked apples flavored with cinnamon and nutmeg are topped with a crispy oat and almond crumble for a comforting and nutritious dessert option.
- **Dark Chocolate Bark:** Rich dark chocolate studded with toasted nuts, dried fruits, and a sprinkle of sea salt, this decadent and antioxidant-rich treat will satisfy any sweet tooth.

- **Coconut Chia Pudding:** A creamy coconut chia pudding made with coconut milk, chia seeds, and vanilla extract, served with fresh berries and toasted coconut flakes, is a refreshing and nutritious dessert.

Seniors can satisfy cravings while supporting gallbladder health and overall well-being by eating wholesome ingredients and indulging mindfully.

In Chapter 4, seniors are invited on a culinary journey filled with tantalizing recipes designed to support gallbladder health, promote digestive harmony, and delight the senses with nutritious goodness. Seniors can enjoy the joys of culinary creativity while also nourishing their bodies with the nourishing goodness of delicious recipes by trying a variety of appetizers, soups, salads, main courses, side dishes, sauces, dressings, condiments, and sweet treats.

This chapter offers seniors a wide range of delicious recipes for appetizers, soups, salads, main courses, side dishes, sauces, dressings, condiments, and sweet treats, all carefully crafted to promote gallbladder health and digestive harmony. Seniors can explore the diverse range of culinary creations offered in this chapter.

CHAPTER 5

Meal Planning and Sample Menus

Meal planning is the foundation of culinary success, providing structure, direction, and inspiration for seniors who want to nourish their bodies with nutritious meals that promote gallbladder health and overall well-being. This chapter serves as a road map, providing seniors with a variety of meal plans and sample menus that are tailored to their specific dietary needs, preferences, and lifestyle.

5.1 One-Week Meal Plan for Gallbladder Health

This comprehensive meal plan is designed to support gallbladder health and promote digestive harmony. Each day includes a well-balanced selection of nutrient-rich meals and snacks that tantalize the taste buds while nourishing the body with whole foods.

Day 1:

Breakfast: Greek yogurt parfait with granola and mixed berries.
Lunch: Quinoa salad with diced veggies, chickpeas, and lemon vinaigrette dressing.
Dinner: Baked lemon herb chicken with roasted vegetables and quinoa.
Snack: Sliced apples and almond butter.

Day 2:

Breakfast: A vegetable omelet with spinach, tomatoes, and feta cheese.
Lunch: Kale Caesar salad with grilled chicken breast and whole-grain croutons.
Dinner: Vegetable stir-fry with tofu on brown rice.
Snack: Greek yogurt, honey, and sliced almonds.

Day 3:

Breakfast: oatmeal with banana slices, walnuts, and a drizzle of honey.
Lunch: Chickpea-quinoa salad with cherry tomatoes, cucumbers, and feta cheese.
Dinner: Grilled salmon with mango salsa, steamed broccoli, and quinoa.
Snack: carrot sticks and hummus.

Day 4:

Breakfast: whole-grain toast topped with avocado and poached eggs.
Lunch: lentil soup with mixed vegetables and whole-grain bread.
Dinner: Turkey meatballs in marinara sauce served over zucchini noodles.
Snack: a mixture of nuts and dried fruits.

Day 5:

Breakfast: A smoothie with spinach, banana, almond milk, and protein powder.

Lunch: A Greek salad with cucumbers, tomatoes, olives, feta cheese, and grilled chicken.

Dinner: Vegetable curry with chickpeas over brown rice.

Snack: Cottage cheese and pineapple chunks.

Day 6:

Breakfast: a breakfast burrito made with scrambled eggs, black beans, avocado, and salsa.

Lunch: a caprese salad with sliced tomatoes, fresh mozzarella, basil, and balsamic glaze.

Dinner: Baked cod with roasted vegetables and quinoa.

Snack: whole-grain crackers and cheese.

Day 7:

Breakfast: Chia seed pudding with mixed berries and toasted coconut flakes.

Lunch: Tuna salad with mixed greens, cucumber, tomato, and balsamic vinaigrette dressing.

Dinner: Vegetable lasagna with whole-grain pasta and a side salad.

Snack: frozen grapes.

This one-week meal plan allows seniors to enjoy a variety of nutrient-rich meals and snacks that support gallbladder health, promote digestive harmony, and delight the palate with delicious flavors and textures.

5.2 Creating Meal Plans with Dietary Preferences and Restrictions

Meal planning is a highly customizable endeavor that enables seniors to tailor their menus to their specific dietary preferences, restrictions, and lifestyle requirements. Seniors who follow a vegetarian, gluten-free, or low-carb diet can customize meal plans to meet their specific culinary preferences and nutritional needs.

Vegetarian Menu Plan

Breakfast: overnight oats with almond milk, chia seeds, and mixed berries.
Lunch: Chickpea salad with diced veggies, quinoa, and lemon tahini dressing.
Dinner: grilled portobello mushrooms, roasted vegetables, and brown rice.
Snack: cucumber slices with tzatziki sauce.

Gluten-Free Menu Plan

Breakfast: scrambled eggs with sautéed spinach on gluten-free toast.
Lunch: Quinoa tabbouleh salad with cucumber, tomato, parsley, and lemon dressing.
Dinner: Baked chicken thighs with steamed broccoli and mashed cauliflower.
Snack: rice cakes with almond butter and sliced strawberries.

Low-Carb Meal Plan

Breakfast: spinach and feta crustless quiche.
Lunch: Cobb salad with mixed greens, grilled chicken, avocado, bacon, and hard-boiled eggs.
Dinner: Grilled shrimp skewers, grilled vegetables, and a salad.
Snack: celery sticks with cream cheese and smoked salmon.

Seniors can enjoy a diverse range of nutrient-rich meals that support gallbladder health while also meeting their individual needs and preferences by tailoring meal plans to their dietary preferences and restrictions.

5.3 Dining Out Tips for Seniors With Gallbladder Issues

Navigating restaurant menus can be difficult for seniors with gallbladder issues, but with careful planning and awareness, dining out can still be a pleasant experience. Senior citizens are encouraged to:

Review Menus in Advance: Before dining out, seniors can look through restaurant menus online to find gallbladder-friendly options and make informed decisions.

Ask for Modifications: Seniors can request changes to dishes, such as swapping fried sides for steamed vegetables or requesting dressings and sauces on the side.

Choose Grilled or Baked Options: Choosing grilled or baked dishes over fried or sautéed ones can help reduce excess fat and put less strain on the gallbladder.

Practice Portion Control: Seniors can practice portion control by sharing a meal with a dining companion or requesting a half-portion.

Seniors who follow these dining-out tips can enjoy delicious meals at restaurants while also supporting gallbladder health and promoting digestive harmony.

In Chapter 5, seniors are given a variety of meal plans, sample menus, and dining-out tips that are intended to improve gallbladder health, promote digestive harmony, and accommodate dietary preferences and restrictions. Following these guidelines allows seniors to eat a variety of nutrient-rich meals that nourish the body while also delighting the palate with delicious flavors and textures.

This chapter provides seniors with a variety of meal plans and sample menus that are tailored to their specific dietary needs, preferences, and lifestyle. Seniors who follow these meal plans and dining out tips can enjoy a variety of nutrient-rich meals that support gallbladder health, promote digestive harmony, and accommodate individual dietary preferences and restrictions.

CHAPTER 6

How to Shop and Cook for Gallbladder Health

Starting a journey toward gallbladder health requires more than just intention; it also necessitates practical knowledge and actionable strategies for confidently navigating grocery aisles and wielding culinary prowess in the kitchen. This chapter serves as a guide, providing seniors with invaluable tips and techniques for shopping wisely and preparing delicious meals that promote gallbladder health and digestive harmony.

6.1 Smart Shopping Strategies

Grocery shopping is the first step toward culinary success, allowing seniors to choose nutrient-dense ingredients that nourish the body and promote gallbladder health. Smart shopping strategies include the following:

Plan Ahead: Before going to the grocery store, seniors can plan their weekly meals, make a shopping list, and prioritize nutrient-dense ingredients like fruits, vegetables, lean proteins, and whole grains.

Read Labels: Seniors should carefully read food labels to find hidden sources of saturated and trans fats, added sugars, and artificial additives that can worsen gallbladder symptoms.

Shop the Perimeter: The perimeter of the grocery store usually contains fresh produce, lean meats, dairy products, and whole grains, whereas processed and packaged foods are usually found in the center aisles. Seniors can shop along the perimeter to prioritize whole, unprocessed foods.

Choose Fresh and Seasonal: Choosing fresh, seasonal produce not only improves flavor and nutritional value but also benefits local farmers and reduces environmental impact.

Stock Up on Staples: Seniors can keep a well-stocked pantry with staple ingredients like whole grains, canned beans, dried herbs and spices, and healthy cooking oils, ensuring they always have the building blocks for nutritious meals on hand.

Seniors who use smart shopping strategies can fill their carts with nutrient-dense ingredients that nourish the body, support gallbladder health, and lay the groundwork for culinary success in the kitchen.

6.2 Meal Preparation Made Easy

Meal preparation is the key to culinary success, allowing seniors to streamline their cooking process, save time and energy, and eat delicious, home-cooked meals all week. Meal preparation tips include:

Batch Cooking: Seniors can prepare large batches of staple ingredients like grains, proteins, and vegetables at the start of the week, making meal preparation easier throughout the week.

Portion Control: Dividing meals into individual portions and storing them in reusable containers makes it simple to grab a nutritious meal on the go while preventing overeating.

Freezer-Friendly Options: Seniors can prepare freezer-friendly meals like soups, stews, casseroles, and stir-fries ahead of time and freeze them for easy meals on busy days.

Pre-Chopped Produce: Preparing and chopping fruits and vegetables ahead of time saves time and effort during meal preparation while also encouraging the consumption of nutrient-dense produce.

Seniors who incorporate meal prep into their routine can simplify their cooking process, reduce stress in the kitchen, and enjoy delicious, home-cooked meals with ease and convenience.

6.3 Cooking Methods for Gallbladder Health

Cooking techniques are critical to maintaining the nutritional integrity of ingredients while also improving the flavor and texture of dishes. Cooking methods for gallbladder health include:

Grilling: Grilling is a healthy cooking method that imparts smoky flavor and caramelization to meats, poultry, fish, and vegetables without the use of additional fats.

Baking and Roasting: Baking and roasting are gentle cooking methods that retain the natural flavors and nutrients of ingredients, resulting in tender and flavorful dishes.

Steaming: Steaming is a gentle cooking method that retains the color, texture, and nutrients of vegetables while reducing the need for additional fats.

Stir-Frying: Stir-frying is the process of quickly cooking ingredients over high heat with little oil, yielding crisp and vibrant dishes that retain their nutritional value.

Seniors who embrace these cooking techniques can prepare delicious and nutritious meals that promote gallbladder health and overall well-being.

6.4 Flavor Boosting Tips

Enhancing the flavor of dishes is critical to culinary success, enticing the palate, and transforming everyday meals into extraordinary culinary creations. Flavor-enhancing tips include:

Fresh Herbs and Spices: Using fresh herbs and spices like basil, cilantro, rosemary, and turmeric adds depth and complexity to dishes without requiring additional salt or fat.

Citrus Zest: Using the zest of lemons, limes, and oranges adds bright and zesty flavors to dishes, increasing their appeal and freshness.

Vinegar and Acid: To add tanginess and brightness to dishes, balance flavors with vinegar and acidic ingredients such as balsamic vinegar, apple cider vinegar, and lemon juice.

Healthy Fats: Including sources of healthy fats like olive oil, avocado, nuts, and seeds adds richness and depth to dishes while also supporting gallbladder function.

Seniors who incorporate these flavor-enhancing tips into their cooking repertoire can improve the taste and enjoyment of their meals while also promoting gallbladder health and overall well-being.

6.5 Mindfulness Eating Practices

Mindful eating practices encourage seniors to enjoy the sensory experience of eating, resulting in a stronger connection with food and improved overall well-being. Here are some mindful eating tips:

Eat Slowly: By chewing food slowly and mindfully, seniors can savor the flavors and textures of each bite while also promoting optimal digestion.

Pay Attention to Hunger and Fullness: To avoid overeating and promote digestive comfort, seniors can listen to their bodies' hunger and fullness cues, eating when hungry and stopping when satisfied.

Practice gratitude: Developing a grateful attitude toward food fosters appreciation for the nourishment it provides, which improves meal enjoyment and promotes overall well-being.

Seniors who practice mindful eating can develop a deeper appreciation for food, increase their enjoyment of meals, and support gallbladder health and overall well-being.

In Chapter 6, seniors are given a wealth of information and techniques for shopping wisely and cooking delicious meals that promote gallbladder health and digestive harmony. Seniors can nourish their bodies with delicious meals that delight the palate and support overall well-being by implementing smart shopping strategies, incorporating meal prep into their routine, adopting healthy cooking techniques, enhancing flavors with wholesome ingredients, and practicing mindful eating.

This chapter provides seniors with a variety of useful tips and techniques for shopping wisely and preparing delicious meals that promote gallbladder health and digestive harmony. By incorporating these strategies into their daily routine, seniors can confidently navigate grocery aisles, demonstrate culinary prowess in the kitchen, and enjoy delicious, home-cooked meals that nourish the body and delight the palate.

CHAPTER 7

Lifestyle Habits to Promote Gallbladder Health

Achieving and maintaining gallbladder health goes beyond diet and nutrition; it is a comprehensive approach to wellness that includes lifestyle habits and practices that promote optimal digestive function and overall well-being. This chapter is a comprehensive guide for seniors, outlining a variety of lifestyle habits and strategies to promote gallbladder health and improve their quality of life.

7.1 Consistent physical activity

Physical activity is an essential component of a healthy lifestyle, providing numerous benefits for both the body and mind. Regular exercise improves gallbladder health by

Promoting Digestive Function: Physical activity increases gastrointestinal motility, which helps move food through the digestive tract more efficiently and lowers the risk of gallstone formation.

Supporting Weight Management: Regular exercise helps to maintain a healthy weight and reduces the risk of obesity, which is a risk factor for gallbladder disease.

Improving Insulin Sensitivity: Exercise regulates blood sugar levels and improves insulin sensitivity, which lowers the risk of diabetes and gallbladder complications.

Seniors are encouraged to participate in a variety of physical activities that they enjoy, such as walking, swimming, yoga, or gardening, with the goal of completing at least 150 minutes of moderate-intensity exercise each week.

7.2 Stress-Management Techniques

Chronic stress can have a negative impact on digestive health, worsening symptoms like indigestion, bloating, and discomfort. Seniors can benefit from stress management techniques like mindfulness, meditation, deep breathing exercises, and yoga.

Reduce Stress Hormones: Mind-body practices such as meditation and deep breathing can help lower stress hormone levels like cortisol, promoting relaxation and reducing tension in the body.

Promote Digestive Harmony: Stress management techniques help to regulate digestive function by calming the nervous system, reducing gastrointestinal symptoms, and improving overall health.

Boost Resilience: Cultivating resilience through mindfulness and meditation allows seniors to navigate life's challenges with greater ease and grace, promoting overall health and well-being.

Seniors who incorporate stress management techniques into their daily routine can reduce stress, support gallbladder health, and improve their quality of life.

7.3 Adequate Hydration

Proper hydration is essential for gallbladder health and optimal digestive function. Senior citizens are encouraged to:

Drink Plenty of Water: Staying hydrated helps keep bile fluid and gallstones from forming, lowering the risk of gallbladder disease.

Reduce sugary beverages: Seniors should avoid sugary beverages like soda, fruit juice, and sweetened tea, as they can cause dehydration and digestive problems.

Infuse Flavor Naturally: Seniors can improve hydration by infusing water with fresh fruits, herbs, or cucumber slices, which add flavor and nutrition without the use of added sugars.

Seniors who prioritize hydration and drink water as their preferred beverage can improve gallbladder health, digestive harmony, and overall well-being.

7.4: Adequate sleep

Quality sleep is critical for overall health and well-being, including gallbladder function. Senior citizens are encouraged to:

Prioritize Sleep Hygiene: Establishing a consistent sleep schedule, developing a relaxing bedtime routine, and optimizing the sleep environment can all help to promote restful and restorative sleep.

Support Circadian Rhythms: Aligning sleep patterns with natural circadian rhythms promotes hormonal balance, including hormones involved in digestion and metabolism.

Manage Sleep Disorders: Seniors suffering from sleep disorders such as insomnia or sleep apnea should seek appropriate treatment to improve their sleep quality and gallbladder health.

Seniors can improve their overall well-being by prioritizing adequate sleep and sleep hygiene.

7.5 Smoking Cessation

Smoking is a known risk factor for gallbladder disease, as it can cause inflammation, decreased bile flow, and elevated cholesterol levels. Senior citizens are encouraged to:

Seek Support: Seniors who smoke should seek assistance from healthcare providers, counselors, or support groups in developing a personalized smoking cessation plan.

Try Nicotine Replacement Therapy: Nicotine replacement therapy, such as nicotine patches or gum, can help reduce cravings and withdrawal symptoms while quitting.

Address Underlying Stressors: Quitting smoking can be difficult, and seniors may benefit from addressing underlying stressors or triggers that contribute to their smoking behavior.

Quitting smoking can help seniors reduce their risk of gallbladder disease, improve their overall health, and improve their quality of life.

7.6 Scheduled Health Screenings

Regular health screenings are critical for the early detection and treatment of gallbladder disease and associated risk factors. Senior citizens are encouraged to:

Schedule Routine Check-ups: Seniors should have regular check-ups with their healthcare providers to monitor gallbladder health and address any concerns or symptoms.

Screening Tests: Ultrasound, blood tests, and imaging studies can aid in the detection of gallbladder disease and the development of appropriate treatment strategies.

Discuss Risk Factors: Seniors should openly discuss their medical history, lifestyle factors, and any symptoms they are experiencing with their healthcare provider to determine their risk of gallbladder disease and the best course of action.

7.7 Maintain Your Healthy Weight

Maintaining a healthy weight is critical for gallbladder health because obesity is a major risk factor for gallbladder disease. Senior citizens are encouraged to:

Adopt a Balanced Diet: A diet high in fruits, vegetables, lean proteins, and whole grains can help seniors achieve and maintain a healthy weight.

Monitor Portion Sizes: Seniors should watch their portion sizes and avoid overeating, as excess calories can lead to weight gain and increase the risk of gallbladder disease.

Participate in Regular Physical Activity: Regular exercise not only aids in weight management but also promotes overall health and well-being, including gallbladder function.

Seniors who maintain a healthy weight through diet and exercise can lower their risk of gallbladder disease and support optimal digestive function.

7.8 Limit your alcohol consumption

Excessive alcohol consumption can harm liver function and raise the risk of gallbladder disease. Seniors are advised to:

Moderate Alcohol Intake: Seniors should consume alcohol in moderation, with a maximum of one drink per day for women and two drinks per day for men.

Stay Hydrated: To avoid dehydration and promote overall health, seniors should alternate between alcoholic and non-alcoholic beverages.

Seniors who limit their alcohol consumption can lower their risk of gallbladder disease and promote better digestive health.

7.9 Maintain good posture

Good posture is essential for spinal alignment and optimal digestive function. Senior citizens are encouraged to:

Maintain Proper Alignment: Seniors should sit and stand with proper posture, with the spine straight and shoulders relaxed, to avoid compression of abdominal organs, including the gallbladder.
Take Regular Breaks: Seniors who spend extended periods of time sitting should take regular breaks to stretch and move around,

which promotes circulation and relieves tension in the body.

Seniors who practice good posture can improve gallbladder health, improve digestion, and reduce the risk of discomfort and digestive disturbances.

7.10 Promotes Social Connections

Social connections play an important role in overall health and well-being, including gallbladder function. Senior citizens are encouraged to:

Stay Connected: Seniors should prioritize social activities and maintain relationships with friends, family, and community members in order to promote emotional well-being and reduce stress.

Join Support Groups: Seniors with gallbladder disease or digestive issues may benefit from joining support groups or online communities to connect with others going through similar experiences and share resources.

Seniors can improve their emotional well-being, reduce stress, and promote overall and gallbladder health by making more social connections.

7.11 Cultivate Mindfulness

Meditation, deep breathing exercises, and yoga are all mindfulness practices that can help seniors reduce stress, relax, and improve their gallbladder health. Senior citizens are encouraged to:

Practice mindful eating: Seniors should practice mindful eating by savoring each bite, chewing slowly, and paying attention to hunger and fullness cues to avoid overeating and improve digestion.
Practice Mindfulness Meditation: Seniors can add mindfulness meditation to their daily routine to promote relaxation,

reduce stress, and improve overall well-being.

Seniors who practice mindfulness can improve their gallbladder health, digestion, and quality of life.

Chapter 7 provides seniors with a variety of lifestyle habits and strategies to improve gallbladder health and overall well-being. Seniors can improve their quality of life by engaging in regular physical activity, managing stress, staying hydrated, prioritizing sleep, quitting smoking, maintaining a healthy weight, limiting alcohol consumption, practicing good posture, fostering social connections, and cultivating mindfulness.

This chapter is a comprehensive guide for seniors, providing a variety of lifestyle habits and strategies to promote gallbladder health and improve overall well-being.

Seniors who incorporate these tips and techniques into their daily routine can support optimal digestive function, lower their risk of gallbladder disease, and enjoy a higher quality of life.

CHAPTER 8

Addressing Digestive Issues and Discomfort

Navigating digestive issues and discomfort can be difficult aspects of gallbladder health management, but with knowledge, awareness, and proactive strategies, seniors can effectively manage symptoms and promote digestive harmony. This chapter serves as a comprehensive guide, providing seniors with a variety of tips, techniques, and lifestyle changes to address common digestive issues and discomfort caused by gallbladder disease.

8.1: Understanding Common Digestive Issues

Seniors with gallbladder problems frequently experience digestive issues such as indigestion, bloating, gas, and discomfort. Understanding the underlying causes and triggers of these symptoms is critical to effective management. Common digestive problems associated with gallbladder disease include:

Indigestion: Indigestion, also known as dyspepsia, is characterized by discomfort or pain in the upper abdomen, which usually occurs after meals and is accompanied by symptoms such as bloating, belching, or nausea.

Bloating: Bloating is a feeling of fullness or tightness in the abdomen that is frequently accompanied by gas, distention, and pain.

Gas: Gas, also known as flatulence, occurs when excess gas accumulates in the digestive tract, causing symptoms like bloating, belching, and abdominal discomfort.

Discomfort: Elderly people with gallbladder disease may experience abdominal discomfort, pain, or cramping, especially after eating fatty or fried foods.

Understanding the common digestive issues associated with gallbladder disease allows seniors to better identify symptoms, triggers, and effective management strategies.

8.2 Dietary Changes for Symptom Management

Diet is important for managing digestive issues and discomfort caused by gallbladder disease. Seniors can make dietary changes to help relieve symptoms and promote digestive health. Dietary changes for symptom control include:

Reduce Fat Intake: Seniors should limit their intake of high-fat and fried foods, as excess fat can worsen gallbladder symptoms and discomfort.

Increase Fiber Intake: Consuming enough dietary fiber from fruits, vegetables, whole grains, and legumes promotes regularity, prevents constipation, and improves digestive health.

Limit Trigger Foods: Seniors should identify and avoid foods that aggravate digestive symptoms, such as spicy foods, caffeine, alcohol, and carbonated beverages.

Stay Hydrated: Proper hydration is critical for digestive health because it softens stool, promotes regularity, and prevents constipation.

Seniors can improve their overall health by making strategic dietary changes that alleviate digestive symptoms and promote digestive harmony.

8.3 Lifestyle Changes for Symptom Management

In addition to dietary changes, lifestyle changes can help manage digestive issues and discomfort caused by gallbladder disease. Seniors can make the following lifestyle changes to improve digestive health:

Practice stress stress management. management. Techniques like mindfulness, meditation, deep breathing exercises, and yoga can help reduce stress, promote relaxation, and relieve digestive symptoms.

Participate in Regular Physical Activity:: Regular exercise promotes digestive health by stimulating gastrointestinal motility, encouraging regularity, and lowering the risk of constipation.

Prioritize Sleep Hygiene: Getting enough sleep is critical for digestive health because it allows the body to rest and repair, regulates hormone levels, and promotes optimal digestion.

Maintain a Healthy Weight: Eating well and exercising regularly lowers the risk of gallbladder disease and its associated digestive symptoms.

By incorporating these lifestyle changes into their daily routine, seniors can effectively manage digestive issues and discomfort, promote digestive harmony, and improve their overall well-being.

8.4 OTC Remedies and Supplements

Over-the-counter remedies and supplements can help alleviate common digestive symptoms and discomfort caused by gallbladder disease. Seniors may consider the following options:

Antacids: By neutralizing stomach acid, antacids like calcium carbonate or magnesium hydroxide can help relieve the symptoms of indigestion, heartburn, and acid reflux.

Digestive Enzymes: Supplements containing lipase, protease, and amylase can help with digestion and relieve symptoms like bloating and gas.

Probiotics: Supplements containing beneficial bacteria like Lactobacillus and Bifidobacterium can help balance the gut microbiome, promote digestive health, and relieve symptoms like bloating and gas.

Before beginning any new over-the-counter remedies or supplements, seniors should consult with a healthcare provider to ensure their safety and suitability for their specific needs.

8.5 When to Seek Medical Help

While many digestive issues and discomfort can be alleviated through dietary and lifestyle changes, seniors should seek medical attention if they have persistent or severe symptoms that interfere with daily activities. The following warning signs may indicate a need for medical attention:

Severe Abdominal Pain: Prolonged or severe abdominal pain may indicate a more serious underlying condition that necessitates medical attention.

Jaundice: Ye:wing of the skin or eyes (jaundice) may indicate a blockage in the bile ducts and should be evaluated by a medical professional.

Fever: A fever accompanied by abdominal pain, nausea, or vomiting may indicate a gallbladder infection or inflammation and should be evaluated immediately by a healthcare provider.

Unintentional Weight Loss: Unexplained weight loss could indicate an underlying digestive disorder or another medical condition that needs to be evaluated and treated.

Seniors who are proactive in seeking medical attention when necessary can ensure prompt diagnosis and management of digestive issues and discomfort, promoting optimal digestive health and overall well-being.

Chapter 8 provides seniors with a variety of tips, techniques, and lifestyle changes for effectively managing digestive issues and discomfort caused by gallbladder disease. Seniors can improve their overall well-being by incorporating dietary changes, lifestyle changes, over-the-counter remedies, and supplements into their routine, as well as seeking medical attention when necessary.

This chapter provides seniors with a comprehensive guide to managing digestive issues and discomfort caused by gallbladder disease, allowing them to take proactive steps to promote digestive harmony and improve overall well-being.

CHAPTER 9

Gallbladder-Friendly Eating on Special Occasions

Special occasions and celebrations frequently revolve around food, posing unique challenges for seniors who have gallbladder issues. With creativity, planning, and mindfulness, seniors can enjoy holiday gatherings while also supporting gallbladder health and promoting digestive harmony. This chapter is a comprehensive guide that provides seniors with a variety of tips, techniques, and recipes to help them navigate special occasions with ease and confidence.

9.1 Planning for Special Occasions

Planning ahead of time is essential for navigating special occasions while maintaining gallbladder health. Seniors can take proactive steps to ensure they have a plan in place for managing their dietary needs and preferences during special occasions. Planning ahead for special occasions includes:

Communicating with Hosts: Seniors can contact hosts or event planners ahead of time to discuss dietary restrictions, preferences, and any special accommodations that may be required.

Bring a Dish: By bringing a gallbladder-friendly dish to share, seniors can ensure that they have a nutritious option that meets their dietary requirements.

Eating Beforehand: Consuming a small, balanced meal or snack prior to attending a special occasion can assist seniors in managing portion sizes and making healthier choices during the event.

Mindful Indulgence: Seniors can practice mindful indulgence by savoring small portions of their favorite foods while remaining mindful of their overall intake and paying attention to their bodies' hunger and fullness cues.

Seniors who plan ahead of time and are proactive about their dietary choices can navigate special occasions with confidence and ease while also supporting gallbladder health.

9.2 Gallbladder-Friendly Recipes

Gallbladder-friendly recipes can be delicious and satisfying additions to any special occasion menu, providing seniors with a diverse range of flavorful options that promote digestive harmony and overall well-being. Here are some gallbladder-friendly recipes for special occasions:

Vegetable Crudité Platter: A colorful selection of fresh vegetables, including carrots, celery, bell peppers, and cherry tomatoes, is served with hummus or Greek yogurt dip.

Grilled Chicken Skewers: Tender chicken skewers marinated in a zesty blend of lemon juice, garlic, and herbs, then grilled to perfection and served with tzatziki sauce.

Quinoa Salad with Fresh Herbs: This refreshing salad features fluffy quinoa, diced cucumbers, cherry tomatoes, fresh herbs, and a tangy lemon vinaigrette dressing.

Stuffed Bell Peppers: Stuffed bell peppers with lean ground turkey, quinoa, diced vegetables, and spices, then baked until tender and golden brown.

Fruit Salad with Mint and Lime: A colorful fruit salad with a mix of seasonal fruits like berries, melon, grapes, and citrus, tossed with fresh mint and lime juice.

By incorporating these gallbladder-friendly recipes into special occasion menus, seniors can enjoy delicious and nutritious meals that promote digestive health while also adding to the festive atmosphere.

9.3 Mindful-Eating Strategies

Practicing mindful eating on special occasions can help seniors savor the flavors and experiences of the moment while also promoting digestive health and overall well-being. Here are some mindful eating strategies for special occasions:

Savoring Each Bite: By taking the time to savor each bite, seniors can fully appreciate the flavors and textures of their food, which improves their dining experience.

Paying Attention to Hunger and Fullness: To avoid overeating and promote digestive comfort, seniors can listen to their bodies' hunger and fullness cues, eating when hungry and stopping when satisfied.

Mindful Indulgence: Seniors can eat their favorite foods mindfully, savoring small portions and enjoying the experience without guilt or restriction.

Practicing Gratitude: Developing an attitude of gratitude for food and the company of loved ones fosters a sense of joy and appreciation, which improves enjoyment of special occasions.

Seniors who practice mindful eating on special occasions can improve their dining experience, promote digestive harmony, and foster a stronger connection with food and community.

9.4 Hydration and Moderate Alcohol Use

Staying hydrated and limiting alcohol consumption are important considerations for seniors on special occasions, as both can affect digestive health and overall well-being. Seniors can:

Stay Hydrated: Drinking plenty of water throughout the day and on special occasions improves digestive function, prevents dehydration, and promotes overall health.
Moderate Alcohol Intake: Limiting alcohol consumption to one drink per day

for women and two drinks per day for men can help prevent digestive issues and improve gallbladder health.

Choose wisely: Choosing lower-alcohol or alcohol-free beverages such as sparkling water, herbal tea, or mocktails can allow seniors to enjoy the festivities without overindulging.

Seniors can improve their digestive health and overall well-being by prioritizing hydration and limiting their alcohol consumption on special occasions.

9.5 Aftercare and Recovery

Aftercare and recovery are critical components of approaching special occasions with gallbladder health in mind. Seniors can take proactive measures to support their well-being following celebrations by:

Hydrating: Drinking plenty of water following a special occasion replenishes fluids, aids digestion, and prevents dehydration.

Resting: Taking time to relax and recharge after a

Special occasions allow seniors to recover and rebalance their bodies and minds.

Reflecting: Reflecting on the special occasion experience, including what went well and what could have been improved, allows seniors to learn and grow from it.

Seniors can support their well-being and maintain gallbladder health by prioritizing aftercare and recovery following special occasions.

Chapter 9 provides seniors with a variety of tips, techniques, and recipes for managing special occasions while keeping gallbladder health in mind. Seniors can enjoy festive gatherings with confidence and ease by planning ahead of time, incorporating gallbladder-friendly recipes, practicing mindful eating, prioritizing hydration and alcohol moderation, and prioritizing aftercare and recovery.

This chapter provides seniors with a comprehensive guide to navigating special occasions with gallbladder health in mind, allowing them to enjoy holiday celebrations while also supporting digestive harmony and overall well-being.

CHAPTER 10

Frequently Asked Questions (FAQs)

Navigating gallbladder health and dietary considerations can raise a lot of questions for seniors looking to improve their health. This chapter is a comprehensive resource, addressing common questions and concerns with detailed explanations and practical advice.

10.1 What role does the gallbladder play in digestion?

The gallbladder aids digestion by storing and releasing bile, a digestive fluid produced by the liver. When food enters the small intestine, the gallbladder contracts and releases bile into the digestive tract, where it aids in fat emulsification, digestion, and absorption. Without adequate bile flow, fats may not be properly digested, resulting in digestive discomfort and other symptoms.

10.2 What symptoms indicate gallbladder disease?

Symptoms of gallbladder disease can range from:

Abdominal pain, specifically in the upper right or central abdomen
Nausea and vomiting.
Bloating and gas
Indigestion or heartburn
Bowel habits change.
Jaundice (yellowing of the skin and eyes)
fever and chills.

If you have any of these symptoms, you should see a doctor for a proper diagnosis.

10.3 What foods should you avoid for gallbladder health?

To maintain gallbladder health, limit or avoid high-fat, fried, and greasy foods, as well as spicy foods, caffeine, alcohol, and carbonated beverages. These foods can worsen gallbladder disease symptoms and raise the risk of gallstone formation. To promote digestive health, eat a diet rich in fruits, vegetables, lean proteins, and whole grains.

10.4 Do dietary changes help with gallbladder symptoms?

Yes, making dietary changes can often help alleviate gallbladder symptoms and promote digestive health. This may include limiting fat intake, increasing fiber consumption, staying hydrated, and avoiding foods that aggravate symptoms. Working with a healthcare provider or registered dietitian can help you create a dietary plan that is tailored to your specific needs and preferences.

10.5 Are there any natural treatments for gallbladder health?

Some natural remedies that can help support gallbladder health and alleviate symptoms include:

Herbal teas: Peppermint, ginger, and chamomile teas can help relieve digestive discomfort.

Apple cider vinegar: Some people find relief from gallbladder symptoms by incorporating apple cider vinegar into their diet.

Lemon water: Drinking lemon water may stimulate bile production and improve digestion.

However, before trying any natural remedies, consult with a healthcare provider to ensure that they are safe and appropriate for your specific health needs.

10.6 Which lifestyle habits improve gallbladder health?

Several lifestyle habits can improve gallbladder health, including:

Keeping a healthy weight with diet and exercise.
Consuming a balanced diet high in fruits, vegetables, lean proteins, and whole grains.
Staying hydrated by drinking lots of water throughout the day.
participating in regular physical activity to promote digestion and overall well-being.
Managing stress with mindfulness, meditation, and deep breathing exercises.

Adopting these lifestyle habits can help protect the gallbladder and promote proper digestive function.

10.7. When should I seek medical help for gallbladder symptoms?

Seek medical attention if you have persistent or severe gallbladder symptoms, such as:

severe abdominal pain or discomfort.
Jaundice (yellowing of the skin and eyes)
fever and chills.
unexplained weight loss
Bowel habits change.

A prompt evaluation by a healthcare provider can aid in diagnosing gallbladder disease and directing appropriate management and treatment.

10.8 Are gallbladder problems preventable?

While some risk factors for gallbladder disease, such as genetics and age, are unchangeable, living a healthy lifestyle and eating habits can help reduce the risk of gallbladder problems. This includes maintaining a healthy weight, eating a balanced diet, staying hydrated, engaging in regular physical activity, managing stress, and refraining from smoking and excessive alcohol consumption.

10.9 What are the treatments for gallbladder disease?

Treatment options for gallbladder disease vary according to the severity of symptoms and underlying causes, but may include:

Dietary changes to relieve symptoms and improve digestive health.
medications that dissolve gallstones or treat symptoms like pain and inflammation.
Gallbladder removal surgery (cholecystectomy) in cases of severe or recurrent symptoms or complications, such as gallstone pancreatitis or cholecystitis

A healthcare provider will determine the best treatment approach based on the patient's specific health needs and preferences.

10.10 How can I help someone who has gallbladder disease?

When supporting someone with gallbladder disease, it is critical to provide understanding, empathy, and encouragement as they navigate their medical journey. This can include:

Offer emotional support and reassurance.
assisting with meal preparation and diet modifications.
Promoting regular physical activity and stress-management strategies
helping with medical appointments and treatment decisions.
Be a listening ear and provide practical assistance as needed.

By providing support and encouragement, you can assist your loved one in managing their gallbladder disease and improving their overall well-being.

In Chapter 10, seniors are given a wealth of information and advice on common questions and concerns about gallbladder health. This chapter is a valuable resource for seniors looking to improve their digestive health and overall well-being because it addresses frequently asked questions while also providing practical advice and solutions.

This chapter is a comprehensive resource, answering common questions and concerns about gallbladder health and dietary considerations. Seniors can confidently and knowledgeably navigate their digestive health journey with detailed explanations, practical advice, and solutions.

CONCLUSION

Embracing Gallbladder Health for a Vital Lifestyle

As we come to the end of our journey through the world of gallbladder health and dietary considerations for seniors, it's important to reflect on the knowledge, strategies, and empowerment we've gained to support optimal digestive function and overall well-being. Throughout this comprehensive guide, we've delved into the complexities of gallbladder health, examined the role of diet and lifestyle in promoting digestive harmony, and provided practical tips, techniques, and recipes to assist seniors in their health journey.

Reflections on Our Journey

Our journey began with an examination of the fundamentals of gallbladder health, including the anatomy and function of the gallbladder as well as the common conditions that can impair its health. We then looked at the senior's guide to a gallbladder-friendly diet, which covers dietary recommendations, food choices, and meal planning strategies to support optimal digestive function and overall well-being.

Seniors now have the knowledge and tools they need to embrace gallbladder health and live a vibrant lifestyle, from creating balanced meals and delicious recipes to navigating special occasions and managing digestive issues. Seniors can nourish their bodies with delicious meals that delight the palate while also supporting overall well-being by adopting smart shopping strategies, incorporating meal prep into their routine, embracing healthy cooking techniques, and practicing mindfulness eating.

Empowering Seniors for Optimal Health

Empowerment is at the heart of this comprehensive guide, allowing seniors to take control of their digestive health and make informed decisions that benefit their overall health. This guide aims to empower seniors by providing practical advice, answering common questions and concerns, and offering encouragement and support as they embrace gallbladder health with confidence and resilience.

As seniors embark on their journey to achieve optimal digestive health and overall well-being, it is critical to remember that progress is made one step at a time. Making small dietary changes, incorporating mindful eating practices, or seeking support from healthcare providers and loved ones all contribute to a healthy and fulfilling lifestyle.

Looking Forward: A Lifetime of Wellness

As we say goodbye to this comprehensive guide to gallbladder health for seniors, it's important to remember that the journey to optimal health is ongoing and ever-changing. Seniors can maintain their health and vitality for a lifetime by prioritizing healthy eating habits, regular physical activity, stress management techniques, and self-care practices.

May this guide be a trusted companion and resource on your journey to gallbladder health and overall well-being. May it inspire seniors to adopt healthy habits, eat delicious and nutritious foods, and develop a stronger connection to their digestive health and overall vitality.

Here's to a lifetime of good health, happiness, and wellness!

In conclusion, we consider the knowledge gained, strategies learned, and empowerment gained during the journey of researching gallbladder health and dietary considerations for seniors. We emphasize empowerment by offering practical advice and encouragement to seniors as they embark on their journey to better digestive health and overall well-being. Looking ahead, we emphasize the importance of ongoing self-care and healthy habits to ensure a lifetime of health and vitality.

www.ingramcontent.com/pod-product-compliance
Lightning Source LLC
Chambersburg PA
CBHW071054290526
45795CB00004B/1479